Smart Nutrients For Smart Babies

A Nutritional Guide for Pregnant Mothers

by Tony Xhudo M.S., H.N.

What You Eat Can Truly Give You a Smarter Baby!

TABLE OF CONTENTS

Dedication

This book I would like to dedicate to my lovely wife that inspired my to share my wisdom to the world from all my years as a "Holistic Health Practitioner".

"I Love You Dawn"

I would also like to dedicate this to my children, A.J., Michael, Matthew, & Edward, Our daughter in laws Kristen, Alexandra, & Alyssa for being there for me when Daddy needed you all! "I Love You All Very Much" and proud to be your Dad !

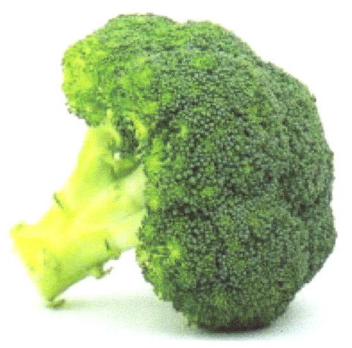

CHAPTER ONE

<u>Smart Nutrients for Smart Baby's</u>
(How It Begins)

It all starts in the brain, safely tucked away in our mother's womb growing and developing at different stage's of pregnancy. During the infant's development stages, it is important for the nourishing mother to provide healthy nutrients for the developing fetus during its growth cycle.

Nutrition, diet, and a healthy lifestyle is one of the most important factors a mother can make for her developing infant, having the most nutritious foods made available to her diet. The effects of brain nourishment a mother can provide for her baby can last a lifetime, and be one of the most important factors in making sure her newborn baby is smart.

As a baby, your child's brain grows at the fastest rate ever. Giving your baby the right nutrition to build his or her brain is critical during her time of pregnancy. Studies done from the Medical Research Council Childhood Nutrition Center showed that infant's who were fed with nutrient rich formula's have the higher I.Q scores than this fed with regular formula milk.

Also those who were malnourished between the middle of the mother's pregnancy term and two years old have brains that are smaller than normal. This inadequate brain growth usually is the result of mother's that are pregnant ,that lack the responsibility in tasking care of themselves with proper food,diet and an unhealthy lifestyle. Alcohol,exaggerates,drugs,and poor eating habit not getting the proper nutrition that is essential in the baby's growth stage's during her term.

This also results in the developing infant to be, having behavioral and cognitive problems throughout the child's lifetime, which includes, lower I.Q. Scores, slower language and learning disorders.

While pregnant, the usual weight gain among pregnant mother's is usually about 25-35 lbs., and on the other hand gaining too much weight also can lead to premature birth's. Also note that premature delivery is one of the greats risk factors for mental impairment, according to studies and statistics.

Diet plays a key role in delivering a smart baby, as I have witnessed in my advice to family members and friends, such as distinguishing smart behavior that normal 2-3 year old's normally don't do or are just not ready for. This I have witnessed many times, advising the nutritional recommendation of what's written in this book for you to follow and comprehend.

Healthy foods that do play a key role in the development of the baby's brain, such as essential fatty acids, DHA/EPA, Fish oils, salt water fish, especially sardines for there rich levels of RNA and DNA factors important in brain growth and development. Fruits and vegetable also that provide the anti-oxidants they contain in protecting the bay's brain from tissue damage during the development stages.

Essential fatty acid's and the omega-3's plays such a profound and significant role in the early stages of the baby's brain development, that will make for one clever and smart baby that will benefit the child's welfare in its lifetime. A deficiency of fatty acid will disturb the development of the growing baby, which is needed in the formation of neuron cell wall and in providing energy for the brain.

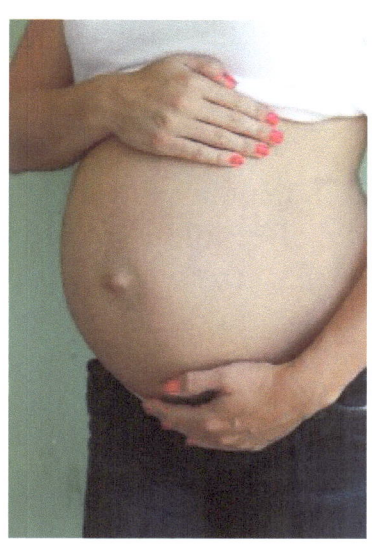

CHAPTER TWO

<u>Healthy Eating During First Stage's of Pregnancy</u>

Smart food choices are the corner stone of a healthy pregnancy in determining a smart and healthy baby. By eating a healthy diet and living a clean lifestyle is one of the best things you can do for yourself and your baby.
After all the food you eat is the babies main source of nutrition, start by making smart food source selections, like switching over from white flour products to whole grains that are rich in essential carbohydrates for a rich source of energy.

You can also get most of your whole grains by providing yourself with hole grain cereals. Fruits and vegetables are also critical components of pregnancy nutrition that provide vitamins,minerals,live enzymes,and fiber. Dark green vegetables have vitamin -A ,iron,and foliate (folic acid) essential to the earlier stages of pregnancy.

Protein, crucial to your baby's growth during the second and third trimester, providing vital amino acid's necessary for brain and skeletal growth.

Fish, being my personal choice of protein has between 15% to 25% of biological value, which means that fish can be used as the sole source of protein in the diet, and for it's essential fatty acid content 0mega-3's. The effect of nutrients contained in fish in the development and growth of the baby's brain is so profound. Studies also show that the building blocks of omega-3 fatty acids,EPA/DHA are critical for optimal brain health and function for all ages as well.

Good Sources of Fish *–are tuna, salmon, haddock, mackerel, trout, herring, and oysters. The deep cold fish, such as* ***salmon, tuna, and mackerel*** *are bursting with omega-3's. Anchovies, sardines, cod,halibut, and mullet are also rich in omega-3 fatty acids.*

Fats build your brain, about two thirds of your is composed of fats, and not just any kind of fats. During pregnancy the mother supplies DHA (docosahexaenoic) and AA(arachidonicacid) to the developing fetus and continues supplying these fatty acids during her breast feeding once the baby is delivered.

Note that the importance of DHA and AA in infant nutritious formula's has been demonstrated many times in infants 10 month's old,that the 3 step problem solving skills were significantly improved.

To build brain cells you need fatty acids,Two of them which are considered essential,the body can not manufacture them and you must get them from food. The first essential acid you need is alapha-linolic acid(ALA) ,which is the foundation of omega-3 family of fatty acids. The second essential fatty you need is linoleic acid (LA) ,which is the foundation of omega-6 family of fatty acids.

Food Sources of (ALA) –*Omega-3; Flax Seeds,Walnuts,Chia Seeds,Green Leafy Vegetables,and Salmon,Mackeral,Tuna,and Sardines*

Food Sources of (LA) - Omega-6 ; include expeller cold-pressed Sunflower Seeds,Safflower,corn and sesame oil.

– **(EPA) Eicosapentaenoic** : Is found in primarily in fish and fish oils.
– **(DHA) Docosahexanoic** :   DHA is especially important to your body ,and is also primarily found in fish.
– **(ALA) Alpha-Linolic Acid** : is found mostly in seeds,vegetable oils,and green leafy vegetables,which gets converted into EPA and then into DHA into your body.

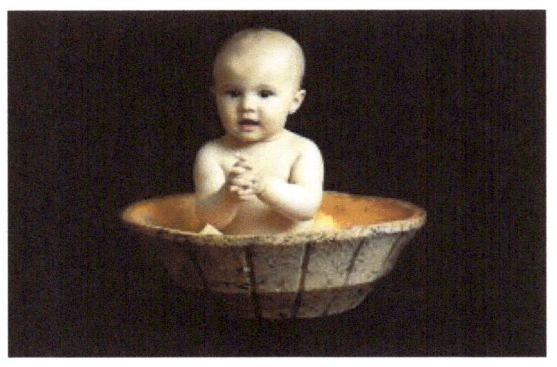

CHAPTER THREE

Omega -3 Fatty Acids During Pregnancy

During the developing stages of your pregnancy,the importance of omega 3's has been acknowledged since the past decade or so ,that omega-3 fatty acids play a significant role in the growth of your baby when it is in your uterus.Omega-3's help to   -

-Build the brain

-Form the Retna's

-Develop the nervous system

-Reduce chances of developing preeclampsia

-Reduce your risk for depression

-Reduce the risk of pre-term labor

So by supplying your body with the proper nutrients and food sources of omega-3 fatty acids,that is has been proven to help you and your baby in the long run.Studies have shown that pregnant women that consumed adequate amounts of essential fatty acids ,their new born babies showed advanced attention spans and greater visual acuity than those newborns that were deprived of essential fatty acids.

During your pregnancy it is especially important that you consume atleast 250 mgs of omega 3's every day,and during the final trimester of your pregnancy it is especially important to during that time of year to make sure your baby uses the omega 3's to for 70% of his or her brain system.
Also keep in mind that when consuming fish,that it can be contaminated with mercury and pcb's.Omega-3 supplements are also available, but make sure that yours is not made from fish livers,as this can contain high sources of Retinol vitamin -A ,which has been linked to birth defects.So omega- 3 supplements should be devired from the body of the fish instead of fish liver.

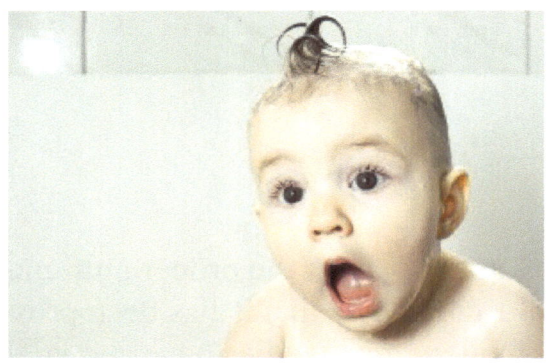

CHAPTER FOUR

<u>Essentiall Fatty Acids & Fetal Brain Development</u>

A recent medical study in Bristol England tracked the eating habits of over 10,000 pregnant mothers on the consumption of essential fatty acids ,and fish oils showed that women who consumed over 340 grams of fish or seafood per week had more intelligent children with less behavioral problems than those that didn't include fish or seafood in their diets.

The latest research also agrees that the omega 3's are essential in the fetal brain development of the child's social behavior.Even beyond the nursing stages it can improve ADHD disorder and other cognitive associations later on the child's lifetime.

Breast milk is also rich in DHA,and it is important that nursing mothers ensure they keep up with their supply of omega 3 DHA in their diet,especially during their third trimester of their pregnancy,and the first year after their birth.

– *first trimester,over 250,000 new neurons are produced by the baby's brain.*

– *by the 6th month of pregnancy the nervous system is developed, DHA accumulates rapidly in the brain and retina,and continues on slowly through the pregnancy.*

- *by the 9th month of pregnancy ,fetal brain development has reached its optimal point.*

Science daily.com suggests that researchers noted that women who ate healthier diets during the pregnancy "per-programed" their babies to later in life seek out foods that to smarter choices in nutrition.

The human brain is compromised of approximately 60% fat and requires essential fatty acids. DHA is the omega 3 fatty acid that plays the largest role when it comes to cognitive development, but EPA also plays a role. Brain size of the baby at birth is almost 70% of adult size of the brain but his or body weight is only 5% of an adult. The remaining 10% of the brain growth occurs during preschool years wherein special attention needs to be paid to complementary foods and micro nutrients compromising of vitamins and minerals.

There is also enough evidence to suggest that foods we eat influence our memory, behavior, comprehension, concentration, intellect, judgment, mood and emotions. There are also 50 brain chemical or neurotransmitters that affected by the foods we put in our stomach.

Smart Nutrients For The Brain

-*Omega 3 fatty acids*

-*Vitamin B-Complex, Folic Acid, cit-C, vit-E*

-*Iron, Zinc, Iodine, Selenium*

-*Choline*

-*Essential Amino Acid's, Taurine*

-*Anti-Oxidants*

Most children that are undernourished are listless, apathetic, and have no interest in normal social activities. The brain being the most active organ in the body and consuming the most glucose and oxygen requires optimal amounts of nutrient dense foods, rich in essential fats,antioxidants,vitamins and trace minerals in order to function at its peak .

Brain Friendly Foods

-*Fresh seasonal fruits, green leafy vegetables*

-*Lentil, legumes, nuts and seeds*

-*Fish, especially deep cold water fish – mackerel, tuna, salmon, sardines*

-*poultry without skin, lean meats & eggs*

-*restrict the intake of salt, sugar by-products, processed foods, and junk foods*

-Ensure adequate supply of prenatal vitamins (if pregnant) and minerals

Surveys have also shown that almost 50% of children that skip breakfast frequently affects physical growth, vigor, learning, memory, and academic performance. This correlates with the malfunctioning of the central nervous system due to various deficiency of micro nutrients. Nutritional supplements to infants and toddlers have been shown to improve memory, cognition and social skills.

Babies have a biological need to constantly learn and any stimulation during fetal life and development, does have a profound affect on brain growth and maturation during the child's preschool years and later on in life. The stimulation of the baby's brain should begin in the womb, it is well known that fetuses do respond to their mothers voices and heartbeat.

The fetus is most alert during the evening hours between 8 o'clock and midnight. It seems that when the mother lies down to rest,the baby wakes up and kicks around. The mother can call her baby and make suggestions or tell stories till she goes to sleep herself. She can recite songs of a lullaby which will all have some affect on enhancing the babies neuromotor development and coordination of the baby.

During infancy and preschool years the mother should interact with the baby as much as possible and should not be left alone in its crib with his toys. Babies learn newer skills through repetition and training till it becomes habitual to them and they find it no longer a need to learn. This interactive play of brain stimulation helps to develop the growth of the child's brain as they are constantly seeking newer ways of learning.

Its been noted that babies love to listen to music, it stimulates the brain in many ways and most children do exhibit spontaneous form of dancing when watching some form of music on TV. As an example.

Conclusions

–   70% of the human brain develops during fetal life, optimal nutrition is required

–   Optimal nutrition for nursing mothers ensures a smart baby

–   Children should be encouraged to consume a brain friendly rich diet in smart nutrients and smart foods.

–   Children should avoid missing or skipping breakfast as it adversely affects growth and behavior.

–   Stimulation of the baby in the womb is equally important to promote brain development by formation of inter neuronal connections, synapses, and dendrites.

The Top 10 Brain Foods For Pregnancy

Eating a healthy diet during your pregnancy filled with a variety of minimally processed foods helps support and ensure that you be providing your baby with brain-boosting foods to heighten their mental acuity.

Green Tea – a powerful anti-oxidant that can help scavenge free radicals that can damage DNA and contribute to many underlying health disorders. A main stay in china and widely popular in the world today as a healthy beverage second only to water. The compounds in green tea can help boost mental alertness and slow down the build up of beta-amyloid in the brain. Drink just one to two cups a day for its beneficial cognitive effects.

Olive Oil – According to the study published in the Annals of Neurology, the monounsaturated fats "the good fats" found in high amounts in olive oil improved cognitive function and memory. So by adding olive oil in our diets that's packed with antioxidants, it will help to reduce the oxidative stress that can damage brain cells, and neuron age related decline.

Flax Seeds – packed with high amounts of ALA-alpha linolenic acid, an omega – 3 precursor that aids in the cerebral cortex functioning better, and in the development of brain cells.

Walnuts – these tasty nuts often used as treats, oddly looks similarly to the human brain. Rich in a host of nutrients that contain vitamin E, folic acid, and essential fatty acids that can have a positive effect on ares of the brain that are critical for thinking and decision making.

Blueberries/Berries-(All) - berries in general serve a wide range of improving functions of the brain. Rich in antioxidants that can help prevent free radical damage that can help prevent inflammation that can lead to brain cell death. Supplementing the diet with berries helps to boost brain cell health that has a direct effect on brain function keeping sharp and mental alert.

Fish – this is no big secret that fish, especially deep cold water fish such as salmon, halibut, and sardines are loaded with healthy essential fatty acids – omega-3's. Studies have shown that people that eat basically any type of fish once a week had bigger brain development in the areas responsible for learning and memory.

Eggs – rich in choline the precursor to acetylene, a necessary neurotransmitter responsible for learning, memory, concentration, and neuromuscular function that stimulates muscles, including those of your gastrointestinal tract. Eggs, also are a healthy way to supplement your diet in benefiting one's brain function.

Avocados – a healthy type of fat that promotes blood to the brain keeping you mentally sharp and your mind functioning at its peak. Did you also know that avacods are a fruit and not a vegetable ? A good source of vitamin E, C,and monounsaturated fat that helps with the reduction of cholesterol in which studies have shown. Used in a mulch-versitle way in many food and dietary dishes,avocados are a healthy and nutritious food that will help benefit the body and brain in many healthy ways.

Whole Grains – are a healthy food source, from oatmeal to whole grain breads
That improves circulation and contains essential fibers folic acid, vitamin E, magnesium, and some omega-3 fatty acids. Whole grains are an excellent choice in addition to healthy diet.

Beets – Loaded with nitrates that can open up blood vessels and increasing blood flow and oxygen to the brain. While eating beets may be a beneficial way of increasing brain health and function,drinking a glass of beet juice may be an even more beneficial way.

Food For Thought

How we think has an impact on what we basically eat, and if your diet revolves around sugar by-products, junk foods, and overly refined processed foods, and saturated fats. Over time, these nutritionally bankrupt foods will rob your brain of the proper nutrients it needs function properly.

By eating correctly with a nutrient rich diet can help your body and brain function to its optimal level. Brightly colored fruits and vegetables provide our body with the antioxidants that protect our brain against harmful free radicals that help improve the signals our brain receives as they talk to each other.

Studies have found that older dogs eating a diet rich in antioxidants were able to perform new tricks and learn newer tasks that much faster than those that were fed a normal diet.

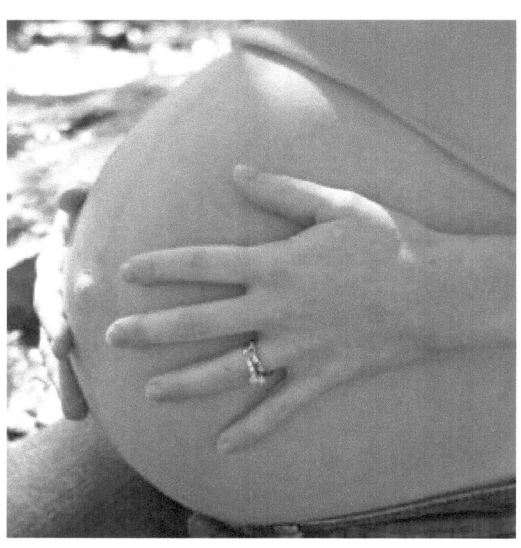

CHAPTER FIVE

<u>Smart Supplements For Kid's</u>

A question that most parents may ask is, should I give my kids supplements?
We are also told that a well balanced diet gives us everything that we need to sustain our well being. In my opinion, years ago as far back say in the 1960's and earlier, may in fact have been true. Through the years one has to take in regard that the top soil in most farms throughout America has been devastated by storms, floods,and hurricane's.

Depending also on what part of the country one lives, eastern coast line, western coast line, and mid-united states, for example those that lived in the mid-united states were deprived of iodine rich foods, and hence hypothyroid and goiter became a common problem for that area of the country. Foods rich in iodine, such as fish had to be trucked over and transported to these areas that had to be kept cold and fresh which often resulted in spoilage.

In the last 50 years has resulted in the destruction of over 50% of our supply of top soil needed for food production and growth. Exhausted top soil that are depleted of the needed minerals and organic vitamins cannot grow healthy nutrient rich foods that we need as a growing society. The human body and brain needs nutritious foods to stay healthy and avoid disease's that were not as common back then when our top soil supply was intact and nutrient dense.

According to the USDA, Americans lack the minerals, calcium, magnesium, potassium, and the vitamins A, C, D, and E. Without these need minerals and vitamins, research has shown that people develop chronic health conditions, and as more and more research and studies have shown, they have linked many of today's chronic illness's to nutritional deficiencies.
Today the press is showing studies that prove supplements with mineral, vitamins, and essential fatty acids do improve intelligence, I.Q., and attention span.

The definition of conventional eating a balanced diet according the (RDA's) the Recommended Daily Allowance has not yet been calculated to maximize a child's mental performance. Today you can find a host vitamins and minerals for children that come in many different forms, from chewable vitamins, powders,gummy forms,canned drinks,etc.

A good source that has been used in children's health trials are, *"Higher Nature's Dino chews".* An essential fatty acid supplement that's often recommended for its purity and quality is *"Equazen's Eye Q".*

The multivitamins packaged for 15 month old's are liquid and if in a tablet they should be pre-crushed and mixed in foods. Gummy formed vitamins are often sold for 4 year old;s and up. One must also remember that vitamins are medicine's and you should consult with your doctor if plan on putting your child on a vitamin mineral supplement,and they should also be placed out of reach where children can not reach them.

Fish oil supplements are generally safe for children as long as they are not taking blood thinning medications, or have blood bleeding problems. You can also buy a gummy-chewable soft type that are a non-fish source of omega-3 fatty acids, as in flax seeds.

Today many of the supplements sold are made of the synthetic ingredients that I would not recommend for my children. The body does not absorb synthetic nutrients as well as natural supplements. So by giving your child synthetic vitamins and minerals, your actually given them half of the nutrients being absorbed. The rest ends up being absorbed as a waste product.

There are now brain supplements for children called *"Brain Strong Toddler " by Life's DHA*, made from algae, a vegetarian and sustainable source of DHA. Listed for ages from 1 to 3 is the first toddler brain health supplement

In a powder form that contains 100mgs of DHA, containing more DHA than any other toddler formula sold over the counter. The powder can be mixed among a variety of foods and is unflavored and tasteless.

The Lifes DHA line of products comes also in *Gummy-Chewable for kid's, pregnant women, and adults. There* product line can be found in popular shopping stores and on the internet.

Protein shakes are a very nutritious way for kid's to get their adequate daily supply of amino acids that are vital for growth that provide a healthy nutrient dense drink, that can also be used as a meal replacement particularly for picky kid's that do not eat a well balanced diet.

Children need protein to help them grow, repair muscle, create enzymes, regulate pH in the blood, control metabolism, and build their immune system. Protein powders come in a variety of flavors that actually taste a lot better than they did years ago. Today it's a very popular way of getting the protein your body requires, flavors come in chocolate,strawberry,banana,berries,peanut butter,etc., so there are a huge selection that one can choose from to suit their taste. They can also be mixed with a liquid base such as ,milk,juice,water,and soy milk,which also provides an extra boost of nutritional value.

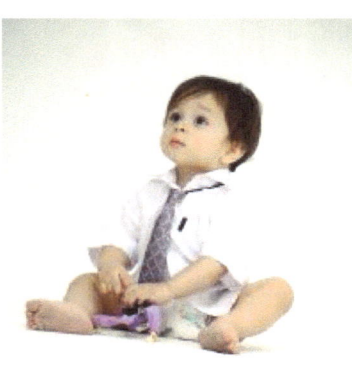

CHAPTER SIX

Which Kid's Need Supplements?

Given the reality of time-crunched parents that generally home cooked meals are not always a possibility, supplements and per-powdered meals do become an option for the well fare of their children. Supplements are exactly that, supplements! Their supposed to supplement your diet with the added nutrition that may be lacking in our diet and one should not solely rely on supplements as an food source:

That is why often pediatricians recommend a daily vitamin and mineral supplement for kid's that are :

Kids who aren't eating regular well balanced meal made from fresh whole foods.

Finicky eaters who basically stick to certain foods that they crave to.

Kid's with illness's and medical conditions such as digestive problems, asthma, or growth related problems.

Kid's that are active and engaged in athletic sports that are demanding on the body.

Kid's that often skip meals, or eat fast foods, and processed foods.

Kid's that don't eat meats, strictly vegetarian, and kid's that drink lots of carbonated sodas that can leach minerals out of the body.

The Top Vitamins and Minerals Required For Kid's

The vitamins and minerals for growing children that stand out and are critical for their growth are:

Vitamin -A – *is necessary for normal growth and the development of tissue's and bone repair, healthy eyes, skin, immune system, and good food sources are;milk, cheese, eggs, cod liver oil, yellow to orange vegetables, carrots, yams, and squash.*

Vitamin – C- *promotes healthy connective tissue, muscle, skin, and also important for growth. Also helps the body absorb iron from food sources. Good food sources are ; citrus fruits, berries, tomatoes, kiwi, and green vegetables like broccoli.*

Vitamin- D - *helps promote bone and tooth formation, helps the body absorb calcium;Good food sources are milk, egg yolks, fish oils, cod liver oil, and fortified dairy products. The best natural source of vitamin D is natural sunlight.*

Vitamin – B's (B-Complex)-*the family of b-vitamins are B1,B2,B3,B5,B6, are required for energy production, body's metabolism, circulatory system, nervous system, and good food sources are ; meat, chicken, fish, nuts, eggs, cheese, beans, soybeans and soy by-products.*

***Calcium – ****helps build strong bones as a child grows to its adult age and good food sources are;milk, cheese, yogurt, tofu, and orange juice that's been fortified with calcium.*

***Iron – ****essential for healthy red blood cells and build muscle. Iron deficiency is a big risk for young girls that begin to menstruate. Good food sources are ; red meats and beef products, turkey, pork,spinach,and prunes.*

Sound nutrition plays a big role in your child's learning and development, so commit to providing your child with best fresh foods possible in a balanced variety of the basic food groups;

My Pregnant Pyramid Guide

– ***Meats & Beans (part of the protein food group)***

– ***Milk & Milk By-Products (provides the body with calcium, vitamin D)***

– ***Vegetables & Fruits (provides the body with vitamins & minerals)***

– ***Whole Grains (part of the food group that provides the body with energy and fiber)***

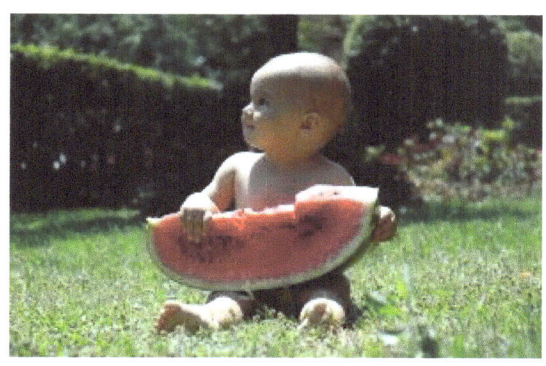

CHAPTER SEVEN

<u>Raising a Smart Kid</u>

There are many advantages to raising a smart child, A smart child that does well in school will have opportunities made available to him or her in getting, scholarships (academic), and end up ahead in many positive ways. A smart kid makes you proud as a parent, and who knows if he/her will be a successful artist, doctor, scientist, professor, or maybe politician.

A lot also depends on his or her genetic make-up and inborn temperament, but genes are not their destiny as well either. By providing your child with the proper nutrients and a well balanced meal as its been written about in this book, you can help your child by increasing her or his chances to be the best of what he or she can be intellectually.

If you are pregnant or planning on becoming pregnant you have the ground work on information to give your child the best chance possible on becoming a smart child and later on in life a smart and successful adult.

The Importance of Breast Feeding Your Smart Baby

It is very important to breast feed your baby after delivery, Mother's breast milk contains vital factors that help with the baby's immune system, provides essential fats and nutrients for the development of a healthy baby.

Another important factor that most pregnant mother's do not know of is their production of a mother's milk called "Colostrum". It's the first milk your breasts produce during the pregnancy that your body starts to make in about 3-4 months into your pregnancy, and may even begin to leak from your breasts during your pregnancy.

The importance of colostrum cannot be overstated and I cannot even emphasize it enough in feeding this to your baby. I can write a book on the importance of the baby's health on just colostrum alone. Its full of antibodies and immunoglobulins that are vital in protecting the new born babies as they come into this world from bacteria and viruses.

Just know that when you're feeding your newborn its first mother's milk, you are basically given him of her their first vaccination towards protection against bacteria and viruses. Colostrum contains over 60 components, and 30 of them are exclusive only to mothers milk.

It is high in protein, fat soluble vitamins & minerals, rich in immunoglobulins, antibodies, that protect them from infections and bacteria. Colostrum also continues to be produced in your body for an additional two weeks postpartum.

The American Academic of Pediatrics (AAP) states that newborns should be fed breast milk for the first 6 months of life, and also recommends if mutually desired by the mother to continue on breast feeding for 12 months or longer. You have to understand as a concerned caring mother to be that human milk is a complex living biological fluid that contains just the right amounts of nutrients, in the right proportions for your baby.

Breast milk features important hormones and special factors that contribute in the health and development of your baby. Also note that preterm milk will differ from full term milk by offering premature babies longer access to colostrum, and higher levels of immunoglobulins and other anti-infective properties.

Studies have shown that feeding your baby breast milk has its many advantages, all the research confirms that human milk protective qualities last well into adult life, and that babies who were breast had a less chance of developing most know chronic illness's and disease's.

The Benefits of Breast Feeding Babies:How they Add Up

By nursing your baby with breast milk you'll provide & benefit the following;

-first milk consumed, is a healthy dose of "Colostrum" (often called babies first vaccine)

-the hormones prolactin & oxytocin are released when you're nursing helping you to relax and stay calm.

– Breast fed babies also have a better chance of not getting sick with less infections and are much more calmer.

– Breast fed babies also have a less chance of getting cancer and major illness's.

– Child that were breast fed long term also were more independent and secure during their growth years.

–   *Lots of research shows that most breast fed babies on their intellectual behavior scored higher I. Q's.*

–   *Breast fed babies receive health benefits that seem to last a lifetime.*

–   *Studies also have shown that mothers who breast fed their babies long term had less of a chance of developing osteoporosis and breast cancer.*

–   *Most breast fed babies were also less colicky during their newborn year.*

Developing a smart begins at birth, by discovering exactly of how we as parents to be, what can we do to increase our baby's chance of becoming a smart baby ?

First and obvious is the planning of having children, then we most focus on our diet, is it substantial enough that I'm providing my baby with the proper nutrients that I'm consuming for my well-being and my child ? You also as must take in the fact that as a pregnant mom,what I'm putting in my body the baby is also. So with that we should eliminate the a lifestyle that isn't going to be good for my baby,like drinking alcohol,reckless lifestyle,stress,drugs,etc.

All these factors do take part in the development of your child, and so many mother's today don't even consider the effect that a reckless lifestyle can do to our baby. Throughout my years as a holistic health practitioner, I've seen many
Pregnant mothers come to me for advice for some other health problem that they were having, and only to remind them that, do you realize that you are jeopardizing the health of your newborn ? And many not being aware the harm that they are causing to their newborn.

So, to me parenting is about awareness of how I can ensure that our baby will be smart and be a happy baby. My research in my life has been spent on private consultations on troubleshooting health related problems that we endure and deal with most of our lives. Most of the literature here that is presented for has been applied and proven to the test with my own children that my wife and I have raised together, and also with many other happy mother's that I have consulted with. Many have also received academic and athletic scholarships because of the research on how do we raise smart babies?

If having a smart baby is your desire and goal, or just having a healthy and happy baby that will have a happy and productive adult life, Here are some tips that you should consider;

-Start changing your food habits and eliminate junk foods, sweets, processed foods, and try and remain stress free during your pregnancy, make sure that you're having fish foods 2-3 x a week or more.

-Exercise is a healthy way to release stress, and maintain a healthy delivery, and it can lower the risk of miscarriage which has been proven to reduce complications during delivery.

-Educate yourself on trying new vegetables, fruits that are healthy for you and baby to be. Make meal planning educational and fun.

-Take your prenatal supplements prescribed from your doctor, make sure your folic acid intake from your prenatal supplements has the required amount of folic acid (.4mgs of folic acid) .Ensure that your diet includes the essential fatty acids which are very important in the development of your baby's brain.
-Avoid harsh cleaning chemicals during pregnancy as they can cause miscarriage and birth complications that can harm the fetus. Be environmentally sensitive and aware of strong chemical odors around you. Stop

-Stop changing your cat liter boxes if you have cats,or just let hubby do it.

-Try and keep a food diary near you to keep track of foods and diet to ensure that you are getting the proper nutritional requirements that you need for your health and baby.

-review the early warning signs of contractions and labor.

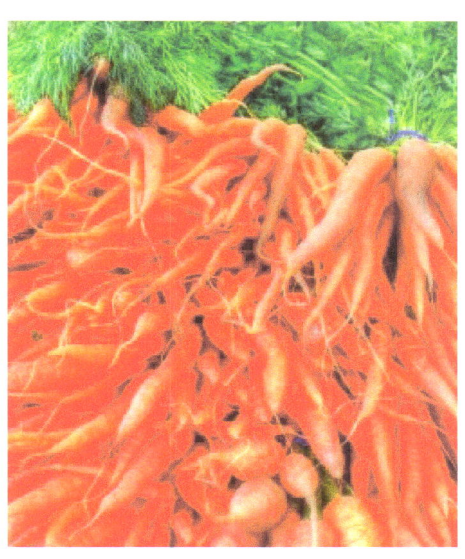

CHAPTER EIGHT

Food Safety Tips

Follow these guide lines to ensure that the food you're going to handle and eat are free germs and food borne illness's as, listeria and toxoplasmosis.

 - *always wash your hands with soap and water before handling raw meats.*

 - *always keep raw meats,poultry,fish from touching each other or other foods.*

 - *always cook meat completely,and under cook poultry and seafood.*

 - *always wash produce before eating.*

 - *always clean your cutting board with soap and water,and lemon Juice scrub.*

- make sure cooking utensils are clean before using.

- do not eat refrigerated smoked seafood like salmon, whitefish, and mackerel.

- stay away from store ready made salads, seafood, eggs, and tuna salad.

- stay away from mercury tainted fish such as swordfish, shark, tile fish or king mackerel.

- stay away from unpasteurized soft cheese feta, brie, white cheese, and blue cheese.
- also note that some herb's can be very harmful during your pregnancy, such as bitter melon, noni juice, unripe papaya, including alfalfa sprouts, and radish.

Women that are pregnant or who are nursing their newborns need 12 ounces
Of fish per week to reap the healthy benefits of fish. Keep in mind also that a low level of fish consumption has been linked to depression in women during and after their pregnancy.

We already know how important it is in eating fish to the development of your newborn's brain development, of how the omega -3 fatty acids are a vital part, as stated many times in this book on developing brain cells and brain power.

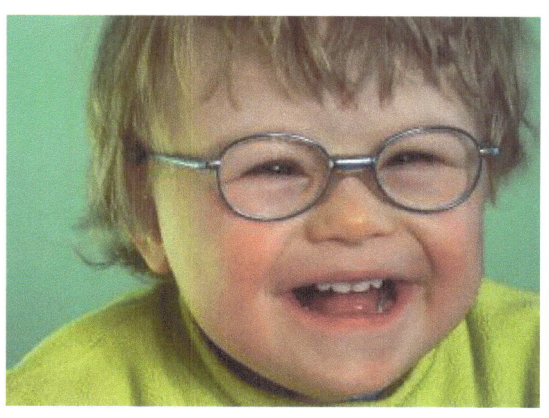

CHAPTER NINE

<u>Eating For Two</u>

When pregnant, women must realize that you basically are eating for two every time you sit down to eat. A pregnancy will take in an extra 300 calories or more a day just to maintain her pregnancy, and the average weight gain among most pregnant women is about 25 and 35 pounds overall.

Those extra calories that you are consuming should come from "My pregnant pyramid" food group – fruits, vegetables, whole grains, fish, and lean meats as stated earlier. By doing so,you are ensuring maximum development for a healthy,smart,and happy baby.

Staying hydrated is also has many vital benefits for a healthy baby and pregnancy, including complications with avoiding early labor, a general decrease in pregnancy symptoms that can become annoying – constipation, swelling, etc.

Drinking adequate amounts of water is important to keeping the blood supply to the babies amniotic fluid. Doctors recommend that you drink 8 to 12 ounce glass's of water a day,and some of the water content your body will be getting will come from fruits,vegetables,and soups.

Typically the human body is composed of about 5 liters of water, but your pregnancy that figure goes up to at least 6 liters, and most of that increase is from blood supply – and blood is mostly composed of water.

An increased blood supply is important as it carries vital nutrients to your developing baby, and also helps to handles the baby's waste products, and toward the end of your pregnancy, your baby is immersed in one quart of amniotic fluid, which is replaced every three hours. You can see the importance water plays during pregnancy and in our health.

In closing I would like to add that, pregnancy is a phenomenal experience to be hold. Don't let the wonder of pregnancy pass you by, as it can become easy
To get lost in the physical discomfort of having a baby forgetting the obvious
That – you are in fact having a baby!

Each pregnancy becomes unique in its own right, as the sheer joy of know that you have together with your partner created life! Pregnancy is the beginning of a life long bond that you will always share with your newborn to be. Ultimately pregnancy is a spiritual bond relating to the existence of "God" that motherhood is one of the most life challenging experience's that a human can behold ! I wish you well,happiness,and an adventure towards fulfilling your quest on Motherhood.

The End..........

www.ingramcontent.com/pod-product-compliance
Lightning Source LLC
Chambersburg PA
CBHW050903290526
45792CB00002B/690